Title page

Fibroptic intubation in thyrotoxic thyroidectomy, a controlled randomized study.

Author

Hala Mostafa Goma MD, professor of anesthesia ,Faculty of medicine, Cairo University.

Coauthor of books.

1-Book published in 2014 in lap lambert academic publishing title of the book is opioid and spinal anesthesia

2-Book published in 2014 in lap lambert academic publishing title of the bookAnesthestic considerations of hepatitis C patients. -

3- Couthor of Topics in spinal anesthesia 2014 in Tech Publisher *Edited by V Whizar-Lugo*

4.Couthor of Diagnostic Techniques and Surgical Management of Brain Tumors

Edited by Ana Lucia Abujamra 2011.

Title of my chapter Anesthetic Considerations of Brain Tumor Surgery

5. Clinical Management and Evolving Novel Therapeutic Strategies for Patients with Brain Tumors

http://dx.doi.org/10.5772/45956

Edited by Terry Lichtor

2. Control of emergence hypertension after craniotomy for braintumor *Neurosciences* . Saudi Med J *2009; Vol. 14 (2): 167-171*

3.Comparison between Prostaglandin E1, and Esmolol infusions in controlled hypotension

during scoliosis correction surgery a clinical trial. Middle East l Journal of anesthesia American University . (M.E.J ANESTH 21 (4), 2012.

4. Control of emergence hypertension after craniotomy for brain

tumor *Neurosciences* . Saudi Med J *2009; Vol. 14 (2): 167-171.*

A dedication:

First of all I will dedicate this chapter for my Great Allah ,
my parents, and to my son Ahmed ,My lovely daughter
Yasmin.

Thanks

Dr Hala Goma

Prof of Anesthesia, Faculty of medicine Cairo
University Egypt.

Table of contents

Abstract:

Objective: The study was planned to compare, the stress response oxygen saturation, the duration of the intubation, and the time needed to evaluate the vocal cords in thyroitoxic patients by fibroptic bronchoscope, Macintosh laryngoscope and laryngeal mask.

Design: randomized controlled study.

Setting: In Kasr El Ani teaching hospital.

Patients and methods:

After patient's consents, 30 (each group=10) thyroitoxic patients admitted for thyroidectomy were included in this study.ASA I, II, anesthesia was started with using 3-5 mg /kg sodium thiopental followed by 0.4 mg/kg atracurium, anesthesia is supplemented with fentanyl 1 μ/kg, intubation in the first group n=10 by the fibroptic bronchoscope, and by the Macintosh laryngoscope in the second groups , Armored tracheal tubes were used in group in third group. The laryngeal mask airway (LMA) has been used with spontaneous respiration and intermittent positive pressure in third group. The following parameters were measured systolic blood pressure preoperative, after induction, and after intubation, oxygen saturation during intubation, and duration of intubation, and for postoperative vocal cords assessment.

Results: in fibroptic group, there was significant decrease of heart rate after induction p =0.001, there was significant increase in heart rate after intubation p=0.000, significant decrease of systolic blood pressure after induction p=0.000, and no significant change in blood pressure after intubation. in Macintosh laryngoscope, there was significant decrease in heart rate after induction p=0.001, and significant increase in heart rate after intubation p=0.001, significant decrease of systolic blood pressure after induction p=0.008.and significant increase in systolic blood pressure after intubation p=0.001.in laryngeal mask group ,Heart rate significantly decreased after induction p=0.021, it increased after insertion p=0.000, and systolic blood pressure significantly decreased after induction p=0.001, systolic blood pressure significantly increased after insertion. O2 saturation during intubation in laryngeal mask group 97.7(0.9), 96, 9(1.3) in fibroptic group, and 95.2(1.6), P=0.004.

Discussion:

The study found that, in fibroptic group, the time of intubation was shorter; the increase in heart rate and blood pressure was significantly lower than the Macintosh laryngoscope, and laryngeal mask group. Although the oxygen saturation is less than the laryngeal mask group, it provided good saturation during intubation.

Conclusion

Fibroptic bronchoscope intubation is better than the usual methods of intubation in thyrotoxic patients especially in the presence of different degrees of difficult intubation, more studies to explain its role in cardiac patients, hypertensive, arrhythmia, with difficult intubation.

KEY WORDS: Thyrotoxicosis, fibroptic bronchoscope, laryngeal mask, Macintosh, intubation.

Introduction:

Graves's disease is an <u>autoimmune disorder</u> that leads to over activity of the thyroid gland (<u>hyperthyroidism</u>, Graves disease is the most common cause of hyperthyroidism. It is caused by an abnormal immune system response that causes the thyroid gland to produce too much thyroid hormone (1, 2). Graves's disease is most common in women over age 20. However, the disorder may occur at any age and may affect men as well Symptoms as Anxiety ,Breast enlargement in men (possible) ,Difficulty concentration ,Double vision Goiter (possible) ,Heat intolerance , Fatigue , Menstrual irregularities in women , Restlessness and difficulty sleeping, Weight loss (rarely, weight gain) .Cardiovascular effects of hyperthyroidism including atrial fibrillation, congestive cardiac failure and ischemic heart disease. Thrombocytopenia may be associated with thyrotoxicosis. Treatment is Antithyroid medications, Radioactive iodine, and Surgery .One of the indication of thyroidectomy is hyperthyroidism that is unresponsive to medical management; recurrent hyperthyroidism (3). The anesthetic challenge during thyroitoxic thyroidectomy confronted the anesthetist is control the stress response during intubation, difficult intubation The anesthetist should expect that 6% of tracheal intubations for thyroid surgery will be difficult (4), and proper postoperative evaluation of vocal cords, to exclude internal laryngeal nerve injury during surgery(5). Fiberoptic intubation is a specialized technique within the field of anesthesiology. The purpose fiber-optic intubation is to facilitate the insertion of an end tracheal tube , into the trachea (wind-pipe) of suitably prepared patient. It might have role in thyrotoxic thyroidectomy in smooth intubation with less stress response .less tachycardia and increase in the blood pressure. Also it may have a role in postoperative evaluation of the vocal cords to exclude internal laryngeal nerve injury during surgery (6). This study was planned to compare, the stress response and oxygen saturation and the duration of the intubation by fibroptic bronchoscope with intubation by the Macintosh laryngoscope and laryngeal mask , and the time needed to evaluate the vocal cords of thyroitoxic patients.

Patients and methods:

After patient's consents, 30 (each group=10) thyroitoxic patients admitted for thyroidectomy were included in this study.ASA I, II. Exclusion criteria were Mallapati 4, coronary artery diseases, congestive heart failure, and atrial fibrillation, obstructive and restrictive pulmonary diseases. The following investigations were be done thyroid function tests, hemoglobin, white cell and platelet count, urea and electrolytes, including serum calcium, chest x-ray and indirect laryngoscopy. A chest x-ray is requested to seek evidence of tracheal compression and deviation. A routine monitors, ECG,noninvasive blood pressure, pulse oximeter, induction using 3-5 mg /kg sodium thiopental followed by 0.4 mg/kg atracurium, anesthesia is supplemented with fentanyl 1 µ/kg, after intubation ventilation was started with rate 10 per minute, and tidal volume 8-10 ml /kg to maintain end tidal CO_2 30-35mmHg. Intravenous fluid of Ringers solution for the deficit volume and the intraoperative losses, careful protection of patient's eyes ,anesthesia is maintained in both groups by 1% isoflurane,muscle relaxation is maintained with 0.05 mg/kg atracurium., intubation in the first group n=10 by the fibroptic bronchoscope, and by the Macintosh laryngoscope in the second groups , Armored tracheal tubes were used in group1,2 , in the third group The laryngeal mask airway (LMA) has been used with spontaneous respiration and intermittent positive pressure ventilation. At the end of the procedure and the resume of spontaneous respiration, isoflurane 1% continued until evaluation of vocal cords in group 1by fibroptic bronchoscope, it introduced through end tracheal tube during extubation, and by Macintosh laryngoscope in group 2, 3. Reversal of anesthesia was 0.06 mg/kg neostigmine 0.1 mg/kg atropine; the following parameters were measured systolic blood pressure preoperative, after induction, and after intubation, oxygen saturation during intubation, and duration of intubation, and for postoperative vocal cords assessment. Statistical analysis using SPSS version 15, Kruskal-Wallis Test, and paired T test, $P \leq 0.05$ considered significant.

Results:

Table 1: Demographic data of both groups.

	Fibroptic group	LMA Group	Indirect laryngeoscope	P value
Age (ye)	40.6(14.2)	36.8(11.06)	43.5(14.3)	0.532
Sex(M/F)	3/7	3/7	3/7	1

In table 1 there was no significant differences in age and sex of both groups. p≤0.05 considered significant.

Table 2: fibroptic group hemodynamic changes.

		P value
Heart rate(HR)Beats /min before induction.	101.7(10.2)	
(HR) Beats /min after induction.	97.7(10.3)	0.001
(HR) Beats /min after intubation.	110.2(8.9)	0.000
Systolic blood pressure (SBP) mmHG before induction.	140.9(11.6)	
(SBP)mmHG after induction	135.5(11.4)	0.000
(SBP) mmHG after intubation.	141.3(10.9)	0.733

Table 2 shows the hemodynamic changes in fibroptic group, there was significant decrease of heart rate after induction p =0.001, there was significant increase in heart rate after induction p=0.000, significant decrease of systolic blood pressure after induction p=0.000, and no significant change in blood pressure after intubation.

Table 3: hemodynamic changes in Macintosh laryngoscope group.

		P value.
Heart rate (HR)Beats /min before induction.	102.2(10.1)	
(HR) Beats /min after induction.	99(10.6)	0.001
(HR) Beats /min after intubation.	114.3(5.8)	0.001
Systolic blood pressure (SBP) mmHG before induction.	141(12.4)	
(SBP)mmHG after induction	135.8(11.1)	0.008
(SBP) mmHG after intubation.	152.3(7.6)	0.001

p≤0.05 considered significant.

Table 3 shows the hemodynamic changes in Macintosh laryngoscope, there was significant decrease in heart rate after induction $p=0.001$, and significant increase in heart rate after intubation $p=0.001$, significant decrease of systolic blood pressure after induction $p=0.008$.and significant increase in systolic blood pressure after intubation $p=0.001$

Table 4: hemodynamic changes in laryngeal mask group.

		P value.
Heart rate (HR) Beats /min before induction.	101. (11.25)	
(HR) Beats /min after induction.	97.9(11.5)	0.021
(HR) Beats /min after intubation.	118. 9(6.4)	0.000
Systolic blood pressure (SBP) mmHG before induction.	140.4(11.6)	
(SBP)mmHG after induction	135.4(11.9)	0.001
(SBP) mmHG after intubation.	146.1 (9.3)	0.004

Heart rate significantly decreased after induction p=0.021, it increased after intubation p=0.000, significantly decreased after induction p=0.001, systolic blood pressure significantly increased after intubation.

Table 5: O2 saturation, Duration of intubation, time for internal laryngeal nerve evaluation of three groups.

	LMA group	Fibroptic group	Macintosh laryngoscope	P value.
O2 saturation %.	97.7(0.9)	96.9(1.3)	95.2(1.6)	0.004
Duration of intubation (min).	4(1.0)	5.2(1.0)	7.3(0.8)	0.000
Internal laryngeal nerve duration (min)	5.5((0.5)	2.4(0.5)	5.5(0.5)	0.000

p≤0.05 considered significant.

Table 5 shows the O2 saturation was significantly higher in LMA group p=0.004, duration of intubation was significantly longer in Macintosh laryngoscope group p=0.000, duration of internal laryngeal nerve examination duration was significantly shorter in fibroptic group p=0.000.

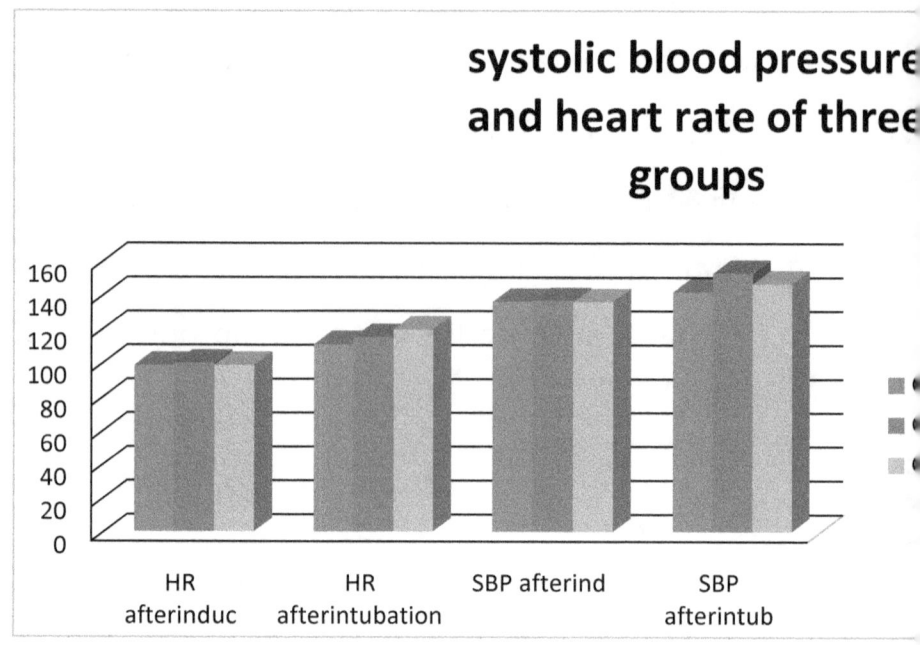

Figure 1: hemodynamic changes correlation between the three group.

G1=fibroptic group.

G2=Macintosh group.
G3=laryngeal mask air way.

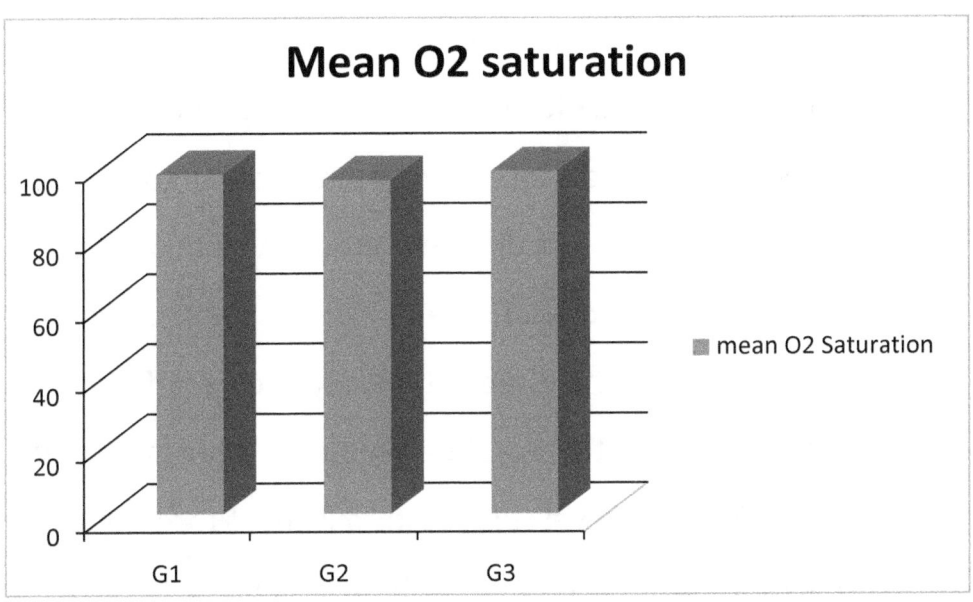

Figure 2:O2 % correlation between the three groups

G1=fibroptic group.

G2=Macintosh group.

G3=laryngeal mask air way.

Discussion:

Hyperthyroidism refers to hyperfunctioning of the thyroid gland with excessive secretion of active thyroid hormones. The majority of cases (i.e., 99%) of hyperthyroidism result from one of three pathologic processes: Graves' disease, toxic multinodular goiter. Graves' disease or toxic diffuse goiter occurs in 0.4% of the United States population and is the leading cause of hyperthyroidism. The disease typically occurs in females (female-to-male ratio is 7:1) between the ages of 20 and 40 years, The cardiovascular system is most threatened with hyper metabolism of peripheral tissues, increased cardiac work with tachycardia, arrhythmias (commonly atrial) and palpitations, a hyperdynamic circulation, increased myocardial contractility and cardiac output, and cardiomegaly. The etiology of cardiac responses is due to the direct effects of T_3 on the myocardium and the peripheral vasculature. In managing hyperthyroid patients for surgery, euthyroidism should definitely be established preoperatively. In elective cases, this may mean waiting a substantial time (6–8 weeks) for antithyroid drugs to become effective. One of the important indications of thyroitoxic thyroidectomy may be failure or incomplete response for medical treatment or the presence of large goiter. Establishing adequate anesthetic depth is extremely important to avoid exaggerated sympathetic nervous system (SNS) responses (7). The great challenge for the anesthetist is to prevent excess cardiovascular activity, securing air way especially in the presence of difficult intubation, and post operative laryngeal nerve examination (8, 9). This study was planned to assess the role of fibroptic intubation, the cardiovascular response, and O2 saturation during intubation, and post operative evaluation of internal laryngeal nerve. The study found that, the time of intubation time was shorter in, high O2 saturation during intubation, the increase in heart rate and blood pressure was significantly lower in fibroptic group. Many studies investigate the role of fibroptic only to exclude internal laryngeal nerve injury and difficult intubation (10, 11, 12) ,but no studies found its role in prevention of sympathetic stimulation and protection of the heart during thyrotoxicosis. the usage of this new technique of intubation may be better in cardiac patients when cardiac stress should be avoided ,more studies needed to evaluate its role in the cardiac patients ,hypertensive patients.

Conclusion of the present study, fibroptic bronchoscope intubation is better than the usual methods of intubation in thyrotoxic patients especially in the presence of different degrees of difficult intubation, more studies to explain its role in cardiac patients, hypertensive, arrhythmia, with difficult intubation.

References :

1. Thyroid Task Force. American Association of Clinical Endocrinologists medical guidelines for clinical practice for the evaluation and treatment of hyperthyroidism and hypothyroidism. *Endocr Pract*. 2002;8(6).

2.Davies TF, Larsen PR. Thyrotoxicosis. In: Kronenberg HM, Melmed S, Polonsky KS, Larsen PR, eds. *Williams Textbook of Endocrinology*. 11th ed. Philadelphia, Pa: Saunders Elsevier; 2008: chap 11.

3.Ladenson P, Kim M. Thyroid. In: Goldman L, Ausiello D, eds. *Cecil Medicine*. 23rd ed. Philadelphia, Pa: Saunders Elsevier; 2007:chap 244.

4. Kahaly GJ, Nieswandt J, Mohr-Kahaly S. Cardiac risks of hyperthyroidism in the elderly. *Thyroid* 1998; 8: 1165–9.

5.Kocak S, Aydintug S, Ozbas S, Kocak I, Kucuk B, Baskan S. Evaluation of vocal cord function after thyroid surgery. *Eur J Surg* 1999; 165: 183–6.

6.Maroof M, Siddique M, Khan RM. Post-thyroidectomy vocal cord examination by fibreoscopy aided by the laryngeal mask airway. *Anaesthesia* 1992; 47: 445.

7.Stehling LC. Anesthetic management of the patient with hyperthyroidism. *Anesthesiology* 1974; 41: 585–95.

8. Brain AIJ. The laryngeal mask—a new concept in airway management. *Br J Anaesth* 1983; 55: 801–4

9.Lacoste L, Gineste D, Karayan J *et al.* Airway complications in thyroid surgery. *Ann Otol Rhinol Laryngol* 1993; 102: 441–6.

11.Wakeling HG, Ody A, Ball A. Large goitre causing difficult intubation and failure to intubate using the intubating laryngeal mask airway: lessons for next time. *Br J Anaesth* 1998; 81: 979–81

12. <u>Randell T</u>, <u>Hakala P</u>. :Fibreoptic intubation and bronchofibrescopy in anaesthesia and intensive care. <u>Acta Anaesthesiol Scand.</u> 1995 Jan;39(1):3-16.

www.ingramcontent.com/pod-product-compliance
Lightning Source LLC
Chambersburg PA
CBHW070756180526
45168CB00004B/1634